Dr Dawn's Guide to Heart Health

Dr Dawn Harper is a GP based in Gloucestershire, working at an NHS surgery in Stroud. She has been working as a media doctor for nearly ten years. Dawn is best known as one of the presenters on Channel 4's award-winning programme *Embarrassing Bodies*, which has run for seven series and in 2014 celebrated its hundredth episode. Spin-offs have included *Embarrassing Fat Bodies* and *Embarrassing Teen Bodies*.

Dawn is one of the doctors on ITV1's *This Morning* and is the resident GP on the health show on LBC radio. She writes for a variety of publications, including *Healthspan* and *Healthy Food Guide*. Her first book, *Dr Dawn's Health Check*, was published by Mitchell Beazley. *Dr Dawn's Guide to Heart Health* is one of five Dr Dawn Guides published by Sheldon Press in 2015. Dawn qualified at London University in 1987. When not working, she is a keen horsewoman and an enthusiastic supporter of children's charities. Her website is at <www.drdawn.com>. Follow her on Twitter @drdawnharper.

Overcoming Common Problems Series

Selected titles

A full list of titles is available from Sheldon Press,
36 Causton Street, London SW1P 4ST and on our website at
www.sheldonpress.co.uk

Overcoming Common Problems

Dr Dawn's Guide to Heart Health

DR DAWN HARPER

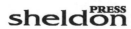

First published in Great Britain in 2015

Sheldon Press
36 Causton Street
London SW1P 4ST
www.sheldonpress.co.uk

British Library Cataloguing-in-Publication Data
A catalogue record for this book is available from the British Library

ISBN 978–1–84709–358–5
eBook ISBN 978–1–84709–359–2

Typeset by Fakenham Prepress Solutions, Fakenham, Norfolk NR21 8NN
First printed in Great Britain by Ashford Colour Press
Subsequently digitally reprinted in Great Britain

eBook by Fakenham Prepress Solutions, Fakenham, Norfolk NR21 8NN

Produced on paper from sustainable forests

Dedicated to my best friend Jack for having such a huge heart and looking after me while I wrote this book

Contents

Note to the reader

This is not a medical book and is not intended to replace advice from your doctor. Consult your pharmacist or doctor if you believe you have any of the symptoms described, and if you think you might need medical help.

Introduction

When I was 12 years old, I was admitted to hospital with appendicitis. In those days, after the operation you stayed in hospital for a few days and, as I recuperated, I found I was fascinated with what the doctors and nurses were doing. By the time I was discharged, my decision was made – I wanted to be a doctor. Three years later, when careers advice was being handed out, I steadfastly refused to discuss anything else. I knew what I wanted to do and, like any self-respecting 15 year old, I knew much better than the adults around me! Finally, my headmistress called a meeting with my parents. She was concerned I was making a mistake. She told them I was a linguist, not a scientist, and that if, jointly, they could persuade me to rethink, I would have a very bright career ahead of me. Thank goodness they failed! I am lucky to love my job, all aspects of it, although I do have to concede that my teachers may have had a point as my working week today involves more time talking and writing about medical issues than it does actually practising them. In fact, when I wrote my first book in 2007, I dedicated it to my German teacher who I still see every year.

So what happened, and how did I get to where I am today? Well, fast forward a few years and I qualified in medicine at Charing Cross and Westminster Medical School. I still remember the day that I called home and simply said 'It's Dr Harper speaking'. I felt on top of the world. To this day every time I drive into London (which is very often!), I look right at the Charing Cross hospital in Fulham with fond memories. After I qualified I spent a number of years working in various medical specialties and took post-graduate exams to become a member of the Royal College of Physicians. I then spent some time working in Australia. They have a wonderful medical system, but it is not *free for all* as it is here in the UK, and, for the first time, I started to appreciate the real cost of treatment and just how wonderful our NHS is. I often say that the NHS is 'like your Mum' – she may not be perfect, but she has your best interests at heart and, one thing is for sure, you will miss her when she is gone. I hope that day never comes, but I do believe we all have a responsibility to look after her.

I have a responsibility as an individual, as a mother and as a doctor and broadcaster, to make sure that my family, my patients, my viewers and my readers are in the best position possible to understand any medical problems they have, and know what they can do to help themselves, which is one of the reasons I wanted to write this series of books – I hope you find them helpful.

For the last few years, I have been working as a doctor in the media alongside my clinical practice. I started by answering medical queries on a consumer health website, which lead to me being asked to write for various magazines and, ultimately, appear on television and radio. In 2013, we celebrated our one hundredth episode of *Embarrassing Bodies*. There have been several more episodes since, and I hope there will be more to come. I am now one of the regular doctors on ITV's *This Morning* and do a weekly Health Hour phone-in on LBC radio. My media work has shown me time and time again that people often leave the consulting room with unanswered questions. Maybe you forgot to ask, or maybe there simply wasn't enough time, and I guess that is the other reason for the Dr Dawn Guides. My aim for these books is to address all those unanswered questions.

In 2014, I lost a dear medical school friend to heart disease. Apart from the fact he was a middle-aged man, he had no risk factors. He had never smoked, and was slim and fit. In fact, he was training for a triathlon when he collapsed and was admitted to an intensive care unit that he had previously worked on. A week later his colleagues and family had to make the awful decision to turn off the life support machine. He has left a wife without a husband, and two children without a dad. It's a story that we hear less often than we did 20 years ago, but it's a story that no one wants to hear. Sadly, heart disease is still the biggest killer in the UK and my friend's tragic story is one of the many reasons I wanted to write this book. My aim is to help you identify any risk factors in you, or your loved ones, and put you in the best place to understand your condition, to know what to ask your doctor and to know what you can do to help yourself.

1

Anatomy of the cardiovascular system

The cardiovascular system is made up of the heart and a staggering 100,000 kilometres of blood vessels. The heart is the most important muscle in the body – without it we die. The heart contracts over 100,000 times a day, pumping over 7,000 litres of blood around our bodies. In fact, the work that the heart does every day is equivalent to lifting a kilogram weight to twice the height of Mount Everest – and it does all that without any conscious effort on our part. If you could buy a pump like that you would have value for money – whatever you paid for it! So, let's take a closer look at the anatomy of our cardiovascular system (see Figure 1).

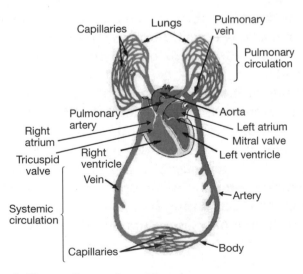

Figure 1 The cardiovascular system

The heart

The heart is basically a four-chambered muscular pump, which sits to the left side of the chest so that about two-thirds is on the left and one-third to the right of the midline of the chest. Very rarely, babies are born with the heart on the right side of the chest. This is called **dextrocardia** and, if it occurs on its own with no other cardiac malformations, it is possible to go through life and never know or for it only to be detected if a doctor is examining your chest and finds that the main pulsation of the heart (the apex beat) is felt on the right and not the left side of the chest.

The four chambers of the heart are two atria and two ventricles. Blood is received into the atria and then passed through valves into the ventricles to be pumped around the body. The left atrium receives blood from the lungs. This blood is loaded with oxygen and is called **oxygenated blood**. Once the atrium is full it contracts to push blood through the mitral valve into the left ventricle. The left ventricle is relaxed at this stage to allow the chamber to fill – this is called **diastole**. When the left ventricle is full it contracts, pumping blood out into the aorta and round the body to all the organs of the body except the lungs. This is called **systole** and the left side of the heart is part of what we call the systemic circulation.

The right side of the heart is part of the pulmonary circulation and is responsible for receiving blood from the body after the oxygen has been used and the waste products collected. The right atrium receives **deoxygenated blood** from around the body during diastole. This is then passed into the right ventricle through the tricuspid valve. Once full, the right ventricle contracts during systole to pass deoxygenated blood into the pulmonary artery and into the lungs.

The aorta

The aorta is the largest artery in the body. It begins at the top of the left ventricle and arches up into the chest before descending down through the muscular diaphragm, which divides the chest and the abdomen and into the lower abdomen. It is 2 cm wide and, in total, it is about 30 cm long. A normal aorta can be felt pulsating in the abdomen in slim people. If the aorta is more than 5.5 cm wide, this is called an **aortic aneurysm** and may require surgery as it could be at risk of bursting (see Chapter 11). Like all arteries, the wall of the aorta has several layers. The inside layer is called the **intima**; the middle layer, which consists of muscle and elastic fibres and gives arteries the elasticity to contract and expand with each heart beat, is called the **media**; and the outer layer is called the **adventitia**.

Arteries

Arteries are the blood vessels that carry blood from the heart to the organs of the body. Just like the aorta, arteries all have three layers – wall, muscle and elastic fibres – to allow them to stretch and contract as the blood pumps through them. The coronary arteries that supply blood to the muscle of the heart are the first to come off the aorta as it arches up through the chest and, after this, various arteries branch off to supply blood to the other organs of the body. Often these are named after the organs they supply, so the brachiocephalic artery supplies blood to the brachial (arm) and cephalic (head) regions, the renal artery carries blood to the kidneys, the ovarian artery to the ovaries and so on. The bottom of the aorta splits into the two iliac arteries, which supply blood to the pelvis and legs.

Arterioles

Arterioles are small blood vessels that branch off from the end of the arteries. They form a huge network and have thinner muscular walls than arteries as they are further away from the heart and, therefore, under less pressure. They connect to capillaries.

Capillaries

Capillaries are the smallest and thinnest blood vessels in the body. They connect to arterioles on one end and venules at the other but, in between, they form a mass of vessels like tiny spaghetti. They filter through the tissues and lie intricately entwined with the tissues. This network of capillaries is known as the **capillary bed**. The huge surface area of the capillaries, and their very thin walls, means that oxygen can diffuse out of the capillaries into the tissues, and waste product can be absorbed and transported, via venules and veins, back to the heart. There are small bands of muscle at the arteriole end of the capillaries that can be automatically contracted or relaxed to allow more blood to be directed to the areas that need it. So, for example, after you have eaten, the sphincters around the capillaries supplying the gut will relax, allowing blood to be diverted to the gut, whereas, if you are exercising, the sphincters around the capillaries supplying blood to your limbs will relax.

Venules

Venules are small blood vessels that connect to the larger veins. They receive deoxygenated blood that is now under low pressure. For this reason, the walls of venules are thinner than those of arterioles.

Veins

Veins are larger than venules but are similarly thin walled as they only have to deal with blood under low pressure. Just as arteries have names referring to the organs they supply, veins are often named after the organs from which they collect blood. So, the femoral vein drains blood from the leg (femur), the testicular vein from the testicles, and so on. Ultimately, veins in the systemic circulation drain into the **inferior vena cava**, which is the main vein delivering blood to the right atrium. Veins in the pulmonary circulation ultimately drain into the **pulmonary vein** and, from there, into the left atrium. Larger veins have valves in them to prevent the low pressure blood from flowing the wrong way due to the effects of gravity. If these valves are damaged, then there is a back flow of blood that can cause varicose veins (see Chapter 12).

Coronary circulation and hepatic portal circulation

There are two exceptions to this pattern of blood flow that have their own special design – the coronary circulation and the hepatic portal circulation.

The coronary circulation

The coronary arteries branch off the aorta and deliver highly oxygenated blood straight to the heart muscle. The left and right coronary arteries supply blood to the left and right sides of the heart, and they drain into a sinus on the back of the heart called the coronary sinus. This then drains directly into the inferior vena cava.

The hepatic portal circulation

The veins from the stomach and gut behave slightly differently to other veins. Instead of delivering blood directly back to the heart, they divert blood, via the hepatic portal vein, through the liver. This means that blood rich in nutrients absorbed from the food we have eaten is directed through the liver so that the liver can use the nutrients and products of digestion and remove any toxins before delivering blood back to the heart via the inferior vena cava.

Functions of the cardiovascular system

The cardiovascular system has several functions.

Transportation A vital role of the cardiovascular system is to deliver oxygenated blood and nutrients to the organs of the body, and to remove waste products and carbon dioxide ready for excretion.

Thermoregulation Blood vessels have the capacity to dilate and constrict. This means that the cardiovascular system can redirect blood to maintain a normal body temperature. In cold temperatures, the superficial vessels constrict to retain heat, while in hot environments blood is redirected to the skin to allow our bodies to lose heat. This is why we notice our veins are dilated when we are hot, but our extremities might look a bit blue when we are very cold. Thermoregulation is vital for life. A 70 kg man running at 15 km/hour will use around 1,100 calories an hour. Without efficient cooling systems in place, this would generate enough heat to raise the body temperature to a fatal 41.5 °C in under one hour!

Protection The blood flowing through our arteries and veins is made up of plasma and cells. Plasma accounts for just over half of the blood volume and is basically the liquid portion of the blood. It is mostly water, but it also contains proteins to help maintain fluid balance and antibodies to fight infection. The cells contained in plasma include red cells that help transport oxygen and remove carbon dioxide, platelets that play a role in blood clotting and white cells that also play a role in fighting infection.

Blood pressure regulation   The cardiovascular system can alter blood pressure in a number of ways (see Chapter 4).

Haemostasis   Haemostasis refers to the ability to form scabs. When the skin is breached with a cut, messages immediately go to the brain to direct blood to the area to deliver platelets to help form a scab. Platelets are usually just circulating and are not active, but as soon as they leak into a wound they activate and become sticky, thereby forming a scab. Without this process, even the smallest wound would mean we would haemorrhage to death.

2

Examining the cardiovascular system

When your doctor examines your cardiovascular system he won't do all the things I am going to mention here. When he takes your blood pressure you probably know a bit about what he is doing, but if you have ever wondered, when you are going for a heart check-up, why your doctor starts by looking at your hands or why your doctor is staring at your neck, then wonder no more.

When I was at medical school, we spent a lot of time doing written and oral exams but we also did clinical exams. Those clinical exams included what were known as **long and short cases**. A long case meant that you had about 40 minutes with a patient to take a full history and do a full clinical examination before two examiners came into the room to quiz you. Short cases involved being taken into a room with half a dozen patients sitting on chairs or lying on beds and the examiners would ask you to examine one small part of their bodies and then ask you what tests you would like to do or what your diagnosis was. So, for example, they might say 'Examine this gentleman's hands and tell me what you think may be wrong with his heart'. And there are times when you really can make a pretty accurate diagnosis of the problems in one part of the body by looking at an unrelated part.

A full cardiovascular examination is rarely done outside medical school, because we use our clinical judgement to focus on the things that we suspect may give us the clues we are looking for. But, to be thorough, a cardiovascular examination involves looking at the hands, the eyes, the neck and the chest, feeling the left side and the front of the chest, feeling in the abdomen, taking the blood pressure, listening to the front of the heart, the neck and the lungs and feeling for pulses in the legs and feet. Please remember that doctors spend years learning how to look for what are often very subtle signs, so if you have a go yourself and think you have found something abnormal, don't panic. It may simply mean you haven't checked properly but, if you have reason to believe there is something wrong, make an appointment to see your doctor.

Hands

Your doctor will look at your hands and, in particular, your nails. He or she will look at the angle of your nail fold at the base of your thumbnail, and will probably ask you to hold your thumbs together with the nails back to back. If you do this, you should see a diamond-shaped space between the two nails. If this space is missing, we say you are **clubbed**. If you have always been like this, then there is no clinical significance to this observation, but if you develop clubbing later in life, it can be a sign of significant disease – including heart disease. Your doctor will look at the nails themselves, checking what colour they are – a blue tinge suggests you are not getting enough oxygen to your extremities. And your doctor will look for tiny dark flecks in the nail, called **splinter haemorrhages**, which could simply mean trauma, but which could also suggest a condition called **endocarditis** (see Chapter 9). Your doctor will take your pulse to see how fast your pulse is going, how strong your pulse is, and to check its rhythm.

Eyes

Your doctor will look at your eyes. If, at rest, you can see the whites of your eyes above and below the **iris** (the coloured part of your eye), this may be because of something called **exophthalmos** and indicates thyroid problems, which may present as palpitations. Similarly, your doctor will ask you to look up as he gently pulls down the lower eyelid to check the colour of your inner eyelid, which should be pink. If it is very pale, this could indicate anaemia which, again, can cause cardiac symptoms such as shortness of breath and palpitations.

Arms

Your doctor will wrap a blood pressure cuff around your upper arm and gently inflate the cuff. When the cuff is tight around your arm your doctor won't be able to hear any pulsation in the crease of your elbow. As the cuff starts to deflate there comes a point where the blood can get passed the obstruction in the cuff because the pressure in the vessels in your arm is greater than the pressure exerted by the cuff – this can be heard as pulsations through a stethoscope. This is the **systolic blood pressure**. As the cuff deflates further to the point where the pressure in the cuff is the same as the lowest pressure in your artery, the pulsations can no longer be heard and this is called the **diastolic blood pressure**. Blood pressure is expressed as the systolic number over the diastolic number; for example, 130/80. It is important that the cuff used is the right size for you. It should cover around 80 per cent of your upper arm. As a rough guide, measure the girth of your arm half way between the elbow and the shoulder: if it is less than 22 cm you should use a small cuff, if it measures between 22 and 32 cm use a medium (standard) cuff, and use a large cuff if the girth is greater than 32 cm. If the wrong size cuff is used, the measurement may not be accurate. Your doctor may want to check blood pressure in both of your arms if he is suspicious there could be a problem with your aorta, as this can show as a difference in the blood pressure in one arm compared to the other.

Neck

Your doctor may look at the side of your neck. This is to look for pulsation in the jugular vein. The jugular vein has no valve between it and the right atrium of the heart, so blood should just flow straight into the heart. If there is a pulsation, this indicates back pressure from the right atrium, which is most commonly due to heart failure but can also be caused by other heart problems. Another thing your doctor will do is listen to your neck, in particular for the carotid artery. Normal flow should not be heard but if there is whooshing noise, called a **bruit**, this implies turbulent flow and could mean that the main artery to the brain is starting to get furred up and needs further investigation.

Chest

Your doctor will start by feeling for the beat from the outer tip of your heart. This is called the **apex beat** and should be found in line with the middle of your collarbone, and between the fifth and sixth ribs. If it is lower than this, or further out, this could mean the heart is enlarged and your doctor will want to check this out. There are also subtle characteristics in the pulsation of the apex beat that can alert us to certain conditions. Your doctor will then place the flat of his hand over the chest wall where the heart lies. This is called the **precordium** and he is feeling for an abnormal thrill or a heave.

Your doctor will then want to listen to your heart with a stethoscope: he or she will listen in different places and may ask you to hold your breath in at times and out at others, depending on what he or she is listening for. Essentially, your doctor is listening for heart sounds and any murmurs, which could suggest damage to the valves of the heart. When you listen to the healthy heart you can hear a 'lub dub' sound. The 'lub' is the sound of the mitral valve (the valve between the left atrium and the left ventricle) and the tricuspid valve (the valve between the right atrium and right ventricle) closing. This occurs at the end of diastole when the ventricles are full. The 'dub' represents the closure of the pulmonary and aortic valves and occurs at the end of systole. If there is a third sound, this can indicate heart failure and a fourth heart sound suggests problems with contraction of the atria.

Your doctor will also be specifically listening for murmurs. As soon as I mention a murmur to a patient they immediately think 'hole in the heart' but in fact this isn't necessarily so. Heart murmurs are relatively common in young fit people, and also in pregnant women, when there is an increase in circulating blood. I have also met lots and lots of kids who have a murmur when they are ill with a fever, only to find that when I check them when they are better, the murmur has completely disappeared.

Legs

Your doctor will start by looking at your legs. He or she is looking for varicose veins and discolouration of the skin, which could suggest problems with your peripheral circulation. If you have swollen ankles, your doctor will gently press his thumb into the skin. If this leaves a dimple it suggests fluid retention. Your doctor will then check the pulses in your groin, which should be strong and regular. He or she will check for pulses behind the knees, on the inside of the ankle and on the top of the foot. Your doctor may press a thumb against the tip of your big toe, which should make the skin blanch. What he or she is looking for is how quickly the normal pink colour returns. If it takes a long while, and if your toes feel cold to the touch, this could mean problems with the small blood vessels in your feet. Just as your doctor listened in your neck, he or she may also use a stethoscope to check for bruits in your groin.

Lungs

Your doctor will ask you to lean forward and may tap your back where your lungs are, listening for a change in the resonance. This is called **percussion**. If your lungs are full of air, the sound should have a resonance to it. If the sound seems dull, this could mean fluid on the lungs, among other things, which can be due to a failing heart. Your doctor will also listen to see if your lungs have crackling sounds, called **crepitations**, which occur when the lungs are accumulating fluid.

3

Tests for heart health

After having taken a medical history from you about your symptoms and examining you, your doctor will have what we call a **differential diagnosis** in his or her head. I was once told, by a very wise professor, that a good doctor spends most of the time listening. By the time your doctor has finished listening, he or she will know what examination to perform to rule out or rule in certain possibilities and by the end of the examination, he or she should know what tests are necessary to confirm the working diagnosis. Below are some of the more frequently used diagnostic tests in the world of heart health.

Blood tests

Your doctor will almost certainly want to do some blood tests if there are any concerns about your heart health. This will involve tightening a tourniquet around your upper arm to allow the veins to dilate. Your doctor may also ask you to open and close your fist a few times to make the veins more prominent. The most common place to take blood is from the crease in your elbow but, if the veins are difficult to see here, your doctor may try from the back of your hand or sometimes even from your feet. Taking blood involves cleaning the skin with a cleansing wipe and then using a small needle attached to a plastic cylinder to puncture a vein. Different vacuum bottles are then attached to the other end of the needle to suck out the blood. Which bottles are used will depend on which tests are required, but common tests would include:

- a full blood count to check for anaemia, which can present as shortness of breath, palpitations or even angina;
- glucose levels, as diabetes is a major cause of heart disease;
- cholesterol, as high cholesterol is implicated in half of all heart attacks;
- kidney function, as high blood pressure can cause kidney problems and kidney problems can cause high blood pressure, which puts a strain on your heart;
- thyroid function, as an overactive thyroid can cause palpitations;
- cardiac enzymes, as damaged heart muscle releases enzymes which we can detect on blood testing.

Chest X-ray

A chest X-ray is taken from front to back. You will be asked to take a deep breath in and hold yourself against the X-ray plate to bring the heart as close as possible to the plate. The films that are produced can tell us a lot about the health of your heart. The heart appears on an X-ray as a white shadow on a dark film, and should be no more than half of the width of the chest in healthy adults. We also look for evidence of fluid on the lungs and other, more subtle changes.

Electrocardiograms

An electrocardiogram (or ECG) measures the electrical activity in your heart. You will be asked to lie still on an examining couch. If you have a very hairy chest, the nurse or doctor may need to shave the hair to ensure good contact with the electrodes, which must be attached to your chest, arms and legs. These amplify the electrical activity in your heart, which is then recorded onto paper. The activity of different areas of your heart is recorded to get a view of the whole heart. It takes about 5 minutes to do and is completely painless.

It is important to recognize that it only gives us a picture of what is happening as we are taking the reading. If you have intermittent palpitations for example, it is perfectly possible to have a normal ECG if it is taken when you don't have symptoms. Other types of ECG measure your heart readings when you are more active.

Exercise ECG

You will be wired up to electrodes and tracings of your heart's activity will be recorded in the same way as for a standard ECG, but you will be asked to exercise in a controlled way on a bicycle or a treadmill. We use something called the **Bruce protocol** where you will be asked to exercise at different levels of intensity. The protocol has seven stages, each lasting three minutes, and each becoming a little more intense up until the last, which aims to get you to reach 85 per cent of your predicted maximum heart rate (MHR). Your maximum heart rate is 220 minus your age for a man, and 210 minus your age for a woman so if you are a 50-year-old man, your MHR would be 220 – 50 = 170. So, 85 per cent of that would be a heart rate of 145 beats per minute. The test would be stopped if the doctor was concerned about changes on your ECG or if you are unable to tolerate it any further. There is also a less strenuous version, referred to as the **modified Bruce**.

Ambulatory ECG

You will be wired up in the same way, but will be asked to go away and go about your normal day to day activities for 24 or 48 hours, while wired up. This test is particularly useful if you have intermittent symptoms, and your doctor may ask you to try to do some of the things that trigger your symptoms. The idea is that you keep a record of when you experienced symptoms. The analysts will look at all of the recording but will pay particular attention to when you had symptoms.

You will be encouraged to keep the monitor on at all times, even when in bed, but not when in a shower or bath.

Ambulatory blood pressure monitoring

This is a very useful test as it gives us a clear idea of what is happening to your blood pressure as you go about your normal day. I can't tell you how often I see people who have high blood pressure when they come to see me, but recordings on a home monitor show their blood pressure is fine. I like to think that is not because I am particularly scary, it's just that they are subconsciously nervous that I might impart bad news and, therefore, are feeling anxious – which puts blood pressure up. If an individual's home-monitored blood pressure is consistently low, and as long as the readings on the monitor correlate with mine, than I am happy to use those readings and we record them in the notes. So, I ask the patient to bring their monitor into surgery. If that monitor shows a high reading in the consulting room, we know the home readings can be relied on. The ambulatory monitor works on a similar theory. You have a cuff wrapped around your arm, which is attached to a monitor worn as a belt, and you wear it constantly for 24 hours (although not in the bath or shower). The cuff will be set to go off a couple of times an hour during the day and just once an hour throughout the night, which gives a good selection of readings of what your blood pressure is doing throughout the day and night.

Echocardiogram

This is often shortened and referred to simply as an 'echo'. It is actually an ultrasound test of your heart. You will be asked to lie on a couch and lubricating jelly will be placed on your chest. A probe is then passed over your chest wall emitting painless ultrasound waves, which bounce back off the heart and give a real-time picture of the structure and function of the heart. It is particularly useful in detecting problems with valves or the function of the heart muscle. There are various options: a **Doppler echo** looks specifically at blood flow through the heart; a **stress echo** looks at how the heart functions when you are exercising. A very specific echo, called a **transoesophageal echo**, involves you swallowing a small probe to have a more accurate look at the heart. This is generally used if you are being considered for surgery.

Myocardial perfusion scan

The **myocardial perfusion scan**, also sometimes called a **MIBI scan** or a **thallium scan**, involves injecting a small amount of radioactive chemical into a vein. This is taken up into the blood stream and delivered to the heart. A special camera is used to detect how well the chemical is taken up by the heart muscle. Good blood flow means good uptake, and registers as red on the monitor. Poor blood flow, on the other hand, registers as blue areas. You may be asked to have this type of scan at rest or while exercising so that the doctors have a clear idea of how good the blood flow is to various regions of the heart.

Cardiac CT and MRI scans

CT scans and MRI scans give a very detailed picture of the heart. The MRI scan involves lying in a tunnel, which is difficult for people who suffer with claustrophobia, whereas the CT scan uses a tube that rotates around you. They are excellent ways of assessing blood flow through the heart and viewing the structure of the heart.

PET scan

This involves injecting a small amount of radioactive chemical into a vein and waiting about an hour for it to find its way from the blood stream into the heart. You will then be attached to an ECG machine and a special computer records all the data as a 3D image of your heart. This gives a detailed recording of the size, shape and function of your heart.

Coronary angiography

This is done to give a very clear view of the blood vessels supplying the heart muscle. A small tube, called a **catheter**, is inserted into a vein in your groin, under local anaesthetic, and then dye is injected. Pictures are taken with a special X-ray machine to watch the dye as it flows through the cardiac vessels, and any narrowing or blockage is then immediately obvious. Depending on where you are having the procedure done, and what they find, sometimes they will pass a balloon through the catheter to open up any narrowed arteries. This is called **coronary angioplasty**.

4

High blood pressure – hypertension

Hypertension is the medical term for high blood pressure. Blood pressure is the pressure created in the arteries as blood is pumped out of the heart. It is usually measured from the brachial artery – the artery that you can feel pulsating in the crease of your elbow – while you are sitting down. It is completely appropriate for blood pressure to be raised when you are exercising or in pain. It is also normal for blood pressure to go up when you are stressed. In evolutionary terms this was a good thing as it is a response to an adrenalin rush, which is part of the fight or flight reaction. If what is making you stressed is a looming mammoth, it's a good thing that you are wired, alert and ready to run or to stand and fight. The problem today is that our stress doesn't come in the form of an occasional mammoth. It is more likely to be produced by the daily pressures to meet deadlines, juggle family and work, and so on, so we are more likely to have high blood pressure for long periods of time.

You can feel perfectly well with high blood pressure. In fact, contrary to popular belief, most people do. People with high blood pressure don't usually have headaches or blurred vision. They have no idea that they are at risk unless they are checked. I think that everyone over 40 should know their blood pressure. I am rarely concerned about a one-off high reading unless it is extremely high. But consistently high blood pressure will put a strain on your heart. Your heart is a bit like your car engine. If you occasionally put your foot on the throttle to accelerate past a 'mammoth', your engine (heart) will cope fine. But if you spend your life with your foot on the floor (stress and pressure every day), eventually your engine (heart) will start to show the strain. That is why we very rarely diagnose hypertension on a one-off reading. If your doctor or nurse notices that your blood pressure is raised, he or she will repeat the blood pressure test once or twice, and may ask you to return on different days, to gather a selection of readings. Many surgeries also use home blood pressure monitors and will ask you to take several readings at home with an electronic monitor at different times of the day to rule out **white coat hypertension**.

What is white coat hypertension?

This refers to people who always have high blood pressure readings when they are sitting in front of a doctor, but whose home readings are normal. The term comes from the days when doctors wore white coats. It is a surprisingly common phenomenon and why many doctors use home monitors or 24-hour ambulatory blood pressure monitoring. If we can prove that your blood pressure is only raised when you are sitting in the consulting room, but that your measurements are fine at home, then it is unlikely that you will need treatment. I generally ask people to take a couple of readings each day at different times of the day for a couple of weeks and then bring those in to me. I also ask them to bring their monitor in so that we can compare the readings in surgery. If the home monitor agrees with my blood pressure readings, then I know I can rely on the home readings.

What is hypertension?

Blood pressure is recorded as two numbers – the systolic value is the highest pressure that system reaches and the diastolic pressure is the lowest pressure. Normal blood pressure is less than 140/90 mm Hg. If your blood pressure is consistently over 160/100, then you will almost certainly need medication. If it is between 140/90 and 160/100 in the first instance, your doctor may suggest some changes to your lifestyle to try to reduce your blood pressure before starting you on pills. If you are diabetic or already have established kidney or heart problems, your doctor will probably aim for you blood pressure to be lower at 130/80 mm Hg.

What causes high blood pressure?

In most cases there is no one specific cause of high blood pressure. This is called **essential hypertension** and is a reflection of how hard the heart is pumping and how much resistance there is in the arteries, which may be caused by narrowing of the arteries. In some cases there is an identifiable cause for high blood pressure, such as kidney disease or hormonal problems and in this case it is referred to as **secondary hypertension**.

About half of all adults over 65 in the UK have high blood pressure and it is more common in diabetics, in people from Afro–Caribbean or Asian descent, or in people who have close relatives with high blood pressure. Being overweight, smoking, drinking too much alcohol, eating too much salt, and being inactive also increase your risk.

Will I need other tests?

If, after several readings, your GP diagnoses you with hypertension, he or she will probably then want to do some other tests. You will be asked to provide a urine sample for dip testing to check for the presence of blood or protein, which could suggest problems with your kidneys. The urine sample will also be tested for glucose, which could mean diabetes. Your doctor will do blood tests to check your cholesterol level, blood sugar level and kidney function and will arrange an ECG to look for evidence of strain on your heart. Your doctor will probably also arrange a chest X-ray to check that the heart is not enlarged.

What can I do to lower my blood pressure?

There are several changes to lifestyle that can influence your blood pressure and could mean that you wouldn't need medication.

Smoking If you are a smoker, you should stop now. Smoking doesn't necessarily cause high blood pressure, but it adds to your risk of developing heart disease. Your doctor and pharmacist will be able to help you with this. Most surgeries now run smoking cessation clinics where you will be able to discuss which methods appeal most to you. Some people use nicotine replacement, others may choose pills to help with the cravings, and some may swap to electronic vaping devices.

Weight If you are overweight, you should aim to lose weight gradually – one to two pounds a week – until you are a healthy body mass index (BMI), which is between 18.5 and 25 kg/m². Even small weight loss can make a big difference – just a one kilogram loss can equate to a fall in blood pressure of 2.5/1.5 mmHg. You can calculate your BMI by dividing your weight (in kilos) by the square of your height (in metres). So, if I am 1.63 m tall and weigh 52 kg, my BMI is calculated as 52 divided by 1.63 times 1.63 and equals 19.5 kg/m².

Diet If you have high blood pressure, it is important that you address your diet and aim to have a healthy well-balanced diet. Watch your fat intake – only a third of your total calories should be fat and you should limit your intake of trans fats and saturated fats to a third of your total fat intake. This means limiting your intake of butter, cheese, pastries, cakes and biscuits. It will also mean getting into the habit of checking food labels for fat content (see Figure 2). This may seem laborious at first but you will soon get to know which foods you should avoid. You should eat at least five portions of fruit and vegetables a day. A portion is a single apple, orange or banana, two plums or apricots, 30 g of dried fruit, two broccoli spears, one medium tomato or seven cherry tomatoes, three heaped tablespoons of beans or 150 ml of unsweetened fruit juice. But, because fruit juice has less fibre

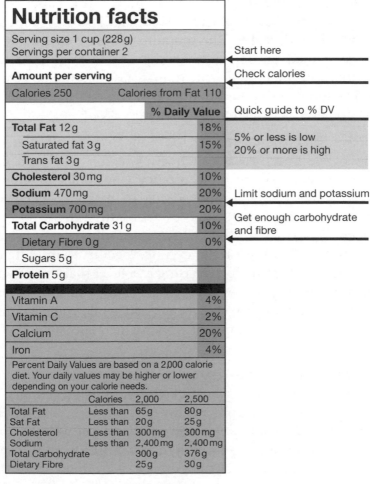

Figure 2 How to read a food label

than fruit itself, you can only count one glass into your five a day. Potatoes don't count as a vegetable in this context. Watch your sugar intake too and beware 'low-fat' options – always check the labels as 'low-fat' often means 'high-sugar'. You should also eat two portions of oily fish each week. This includes mackerel, sardines, kippers, salmon, pilchards, herring or fresh tuna.

Salt We have got used to a high-salt diet in the western world. You should limit your daily intake to 6 grams and, when you start looking at the hidden salt in processed foods, you will be shocked by the amounts. Limit your intake of processed food and try not adding salt to your food. At first this will taste bland, but human taste buds adapt very quickly and by using herbs and spices you will soon wonder how you ever managed to eat such salty food!

Exercise You should aim to do half an hour of exercise at least five times a week. It doesn't matter what you do, and it doesn't have to be in a fancy gym, but you should choose something you enjoy doing so that you will stick with it and, even better, try to exercise with a friend so that you encourage each other when your willpower is weak. So, whether it's a brisk walk, cycling, jogging, swimming or dancing, you need to be exercising at a level that makes you out of breath. If you are gasping for breath, you should ease back a bit but if you can chat away easily while you are doing your exercise then you are not working hard enough and you need to up your game!

Alcohol Drinking to excess can lead to an increase in blood pressure, so make sure you stick to recommended limits of alcohol – that is, 14 units per week for women and 21 for men – and try to have at least two dry days per week. A unit of alcohol is probably a lot less than you think. The simple way to calculate your alcohol intake is by looking at the percentage alcohol in the drink you are drinking. The percentage alcohol shows you the number of units in a litre of that drink; for wine, a 75 cl bottle is three-quarters of a litre (75 cl = 750 ml; 1 litre = 1000 ml), so if the wine contains 12 per cent alcohol, the number of units in the bottle is three-quarters of 12 = 9 units. If you are pouring a glass at home it is likely to be a 250 ml glass and that will contain three units not one.

Caffeine   The effect that caffeine has on blood pressure is probably very small, but if you have high blood pressure then it is a good idea to restrict your intake to five caffeinated drinks per day.

What if I need medication to treat my blood pressure?

If your blood pressure remains high despite changes to your lifestyle, your doctor will start you on pills. There are many different types of anti-hypertensive drugs and which ones you are prescribed will depend on your individual circumstances, what other medications you are on and what other illnesses you have. You may end up needing more than one type of pill. If you develop side effects, always discuss these with your doctor as there is always an alternative, but never stop taking any prescribed medicine without talking to your doctor first. If your heart is already showing signs of strain then your doctor may suggest you start taking a low dose of aspirin and, if your cholesterol is high, he or she may also give you a statin to reduce your cholesterol level. Most people who start blood pressure treatment will need to be on that treatment for life but, if you manage to lose more weight and make other changes to your lifestyle, it is possible to come off medication altogether.

5

Cholesterol

Cholesterol is a fat or lipid, which is partly made in cells in our body, and partly derived from the food that we eat. Not all cholesterol is bad and, in fact, we need some cholesterol to stay healthy. When we measure cholesterol, we measure the total cholesterol in the blood, but we also look at the levels of different **lipoproteins** that circulate in the bloodstream. As the name suggests, lipoproteins are compounds which are a combination of protein and lipid. In other words, this is the way cholesterol, and other fats, are transported in the bloodstream. There are several different lipoproteins but the ones particularly relevant to cholesterol are low density lipoproteins (LDLs) and high density lipoproteins (HDLs). The LDLs are often referred to as 'bad' cholesterol and the HDLs as 'good' cholesterol. The LDLs comprise the majority of the cholesterol. If you are diabetic, or have already been diagnosed with heart disease, your doctor will want to reduce your total cholesterol level, but if you are at risk of developing heart disease, he or she will be more interested in the ratio of your good cholesterol to the level of total cholesterol in your blood.

What is normal cholesterol?

Cholesterol is measured in the blood in mmol per litre. Total cholesterol should be less than 5.0 mmol per litre; LDL cholesterol should be less than 3 mmol per litre; and HDL cholesterol more than 1.2 mmol per litre. Generally speaking, the lower your LDL and the higher your HDL, the better. We often look at the ratio of total cholesterol to HDL:

the figure for total cholesterol divided by the figure for HDL should ideally be less than 4.5. However, whether your doctor decides to treat your cholesterol or not, will depend on other risk factors for heart disease, such as your age, gender, blood pressure and whether or not you smoke.

How can I tell if my cholesterol is high?

Very occasionally a high cholesterol level will cause yellow, waxy-looking plaques in the skin around the eyes, called **xan-thelasma**, or fatty lumps on the elbows, called **xanthomas**. But, in the vast majority of cases, there is no obvious outside sign that your cholesterol is high and the only way to know is to have a blood test. Some chemists offer a pinprick test, which gives you an idea of your total cholesterol. If you have a test like this which suggests your level is high, your doctor will want to do a formal blood test. These are usually done on a fasting sample, which means having had nothing to eat or drink for eight hours prior to the blood test.

How can my cholesterol be high if I eat healthily?

Only about 10–20 per cent of your total cholesterol comes from what you eat. The rest is made by your body, and that amount is genetically predetermined. That is why it is possible to find fat people who eat a high cholesterol diet but still have low cholesterol in their blood stream, and others, who eat healthily, but who have high cholesterol because their bodies make more of it.

Why does cholesterol matter?

High levels of cholesterol can cause fatty plaques to form on the walls of the blood vessels. Over time these plaques can build up and harden, forming what is known as **athero-**

sclerosis or hardening of the arteries, which can mean not enough blood gets delivered to certain parts of the body. If the plaques form in the coronary arteries, this causes heart disease. If they form in the blood vessels supplying the brain, they can cause strokes, and if they form in the vessels in the legs, they can cause severe pain in the legs when walking. This is called **claudication**. Sometimes blood clots form on the plaques and, if they break off, they can block an artery, meaning that no blood can get through and this can cause a heart attack, stroke or gangrene. It is thought that high cholesterol is implicated in half of all heart attacks but, of course, cholesterol isn't the whole story. There are several other risk factors that play a role.

What other risk factors are there for heart disease?

When your doctor is deciding whether he or she needs to treat your cholesterol level, he or she will take into account your overall risk. There are some risk factors that you can do nothing about. These include:

- age
- gender
- ethnicity
- family history
- menopause status.

The older you are the more likely you are to develop atheroma, and men are more likely to develop atheroma than women. In addition, Asian and Afro–Caribbean people are more prone to atheroma than Caucasians. Family history has an effect as, if your father or brother developed heart disease or had a stroke before the age of 55, or your mother or sister developed these problems before 60, then you are at increased risk. The average age for the menopause in the UK is 51. If you have your menopause before 45, this is called an early menopause. Oestrogen has a protective effect on the heart, so going through an early menopause when your oestrogen levels fall early also puts you at increased risk.

However, there are other risk factors that are related to our lifestyles and which we most definitely can do something about. These include:

- smoking
- obesity
- high alcohol intake
- high-fat, high-salt diet
- inactivity
- type 2 diabetes.

Your risks can also be influenced by other conditions such as high blood pressure and kidney problems. The more risk factors you have the more likely you are to develop heart disease.

How will my doctor assess my risk?

Once your doctor has your cholesterol result, he or she will also want to take your blood pressure and will need to know whether or not you smoke. Your doctor will then plot these values on a graph. The graphs have been created after researchers have looked at, literally, thousands of people and worked out the relative risks of each of them developing heart disease (see Table 1).

So, if you are a 50-year-old non-diabetic woman who smokes and has a blood pressure of 120/80 and a total cholesterol to HDL ratio of 4, then your risk of developing cardiovascular disease in the next ten years is less than 10 per cent.

If, however, you are a 61-year-old non-diabetic man who doesn't smoke and has a blood pressure of 130/80 and a total cholesterol to HDL ratio of 6, then your risk of developing heart disease in the next ten years is 20 per cent.

Table 1 Factors linked to the risk of suffering a first heart attack in the INTERHEART study

Risk factor	Increase in heart attack risk
Hypertension alone	1.9 times
Diabetes alone	2.4 times
Smoking alone	2.9 times
Abnormal lipid profile (dyslipidaemia)	3.3 times
Hypertension, diabetes, smoking	13.0 times
Hypertension, diabetes, smoking, dyslipidaemia	42.3 times
Hypertension, diabetes, smoking, dyslipidaemia, obesity	68.5 times
Hypertension, diabetes, smoking, dyslipidaemia, psychosocial factors	182.9 times
Hypertension, diabetes, smoking, dyslipidaemia, psychosocial factors, obesity	333.7 times

Source: Yusuf S, Hawken S, Ounpuu S, Dans T, Auezum A, Lana F, et al. Effect of potentially modifiable risk factors associated with myocardial infarction in 52 countries (the INTERHEART study): case-control study. *Lancet*. 2004; **364** (9438): 937–52.

Do I need treatment for my cholesterol?

Your doctor will advise you to address any lifestyle issues that could increase your risk. So if you smoke, you should stop, and your doctor will be able to help you with advice about local smoking cessation services. You should aim for a healthy BMI of between 18.5 and 25 kg/m². You should restrict your alcohol to recommended limits – that's 14 units a week for women and 21 units a week for men with at least two dry days a week. Watch your salt and fat intake, and try to keep to a low cholesterol diet. You should also aim to exercise for 30 minutes at least five times a week.

Your doctor may suggest you start treatment if you:

- have a 10 per cent (or greater) risk of developing heart disease in the next ten years;
- have known cardiovascular disease;
- are diabetic;

- if you have a total cholesterol to HDL ratio of 6 or more;
- have a family history of high cholesterol.

What does treatment involve?

The most common type of medicine used to treat high cholesterol is a group of drugs called **statins**. They work by inhibiting an enzyme in the liver which reduces the production of cholesterol. You will need a blood test to check your liver is healthy before starting treatment and again, three months later. If all is well, you will just need your liver blood tests to be monitored once a year. Statins are generally well-tolerated but they can cause muscle aches in some people. These are usually mild but, occasionally. they can lead to serious muscle problems so it is important that you report any symptoms to your doctor, who will probably want to do a blood test to check your muscle enzymes. If these are very raised, it suggests muscle damage and your doctor will advise that you stop taking your statin.

There is also a drug called **ezetimibe** which works by blocking absorption of cholesterol from the gut. By definition this could only ever reduce your total cholesterol by a maximum of 20 per cent, but it is useful in patients who cannot tolerate statins or it can be used in conjunction with a statin for those with very high cholesterol levels.

6

Coronary heart disease

The heart is a four-chambered muscular organ that requires a good blood supply to work efficiently. It gets its blood supply from the coronary arteries, which are the first arteries to branch off the aorta as it leaves the left ventricle. If those blood vessels get furred up, the blood supply to the heart muscle (or *myocardium*) is compromised. This is called *coronary heart disease* or *ischaemic heart disease* and may cause symptoms of *angina* or a heart attack. Anyone can have a heart attack, but they are more frequent in older people, and are more frequent in men than women. Chapter 5 gives more details about who is more at risk of having a heart attack.

What is a heart attack?

A heart attack is where the blood supply to part of the heart is cut off, causing the muscle supplied by that vessel to die. A heart attack is also sometimes called a **myocardial infarction** (MI) – myocardial meaning heart muscle and infarction meaning dead tissue. A heart attack, or MI, usually presents with a central crushing chest pain which may radiate into the left arm, neck or jaw. Sometimes the pain is felt in both arms and sometimes there may be no pain but the attack is picked up on an ECG tracing. The pain may be associated with shortness of breath and feeling sick or light headed. You may feel clammy, and those around you may think you look pale or grey. This is a medical emergency and you, or someone near you, should call 999 immediately.

The most common cause of a heart attack is a clot blocking an artery. The size and severity of the heart attack depends on the size of the blood vessel that is blocked. If a small artery is blocked, then a small area of muscle will be affected and you are less likely to have long-term problems. If one of the main coronary arteries is blocked, then a large part of muscle is affected and, unless the blood vessel can be opened again quickly, you are likely to be left very short of breath on minimal exertion because the heart simply can't pump hard enough with the healthy muscle that is left. Heart attacks can also cause abnormal heart rhythms, which can be fatal.

How is a heart attack diagnosed?

A doctor will immediately suspect a heart attack in anyone who has the symptoms mentioned above, and will arrange an ECG. There are specific changes on the ECG tracing that occur when heart muscle is being damaged. Where those changes occur depends on which bit of muscle is being damaged. If an MI is suspected, a blood test will be arranged looking for a rise in a chemical called **troponin**. When heart muscle is damaged it releases this chemical into the bloodstream; it will start to rise within 3 hours of a heart attack. It peaks between 24 and 48 hours and will then return to normal over the next 5 to 14 days.

How is a heart attack treated?

If you have a heart attack, you will be probably be given an aspirin to thin your blood. You may also be offered other blood-thinning agents. If we can restore blood flow to the heart muscle quickly (within a few hours), we can minimize the damage to the heart muscle. If your symptoms are caught early and the facilities are available you may be offered an injection of a clot-busting drug. You can only have this once in your lifetime as your body develops antibodies to it so, if you have had a previous heart attack where this was administered, you will not be offered it again – you may be offered an angioplasty instead. This is where a small wire with a balloon on the end is inserted into the large artery in your groin or arm and then, under X-ray control, is passed into the coronary artery. When it reaches the site of the blockage, the balloon can be inflated to open up the artery again. The doctors may leave a stent in the artery to keep it open.

After a heart attack you will be admitted to hospital where you will probably be looked after in a coronary care unit where the nurses and doctors have special expertise in looking after people with heart problems. You will be attached to a heart monitor so they can monitor your heart rhythm and you will have regular blood tests. Over the next few days you are likely to be started on a combination of drugs, and these may include:

- nitrates, which dilate blood vessels and help maintain a healthy blood flow to the heart;
- beta blockers, which slow the heart rate and keep a steady rhythm;
- angiotensin converting enzyme (ACE) inhibitors, which lower blood pressure;
- statins, which lower cholesterol.

What happens after I leave hospital?

When you leave hospital the hospital will contact your GP so that he or she knows what has happened, and that you are now on a new cocktail of medicines to protect your heart. You will be given a short course of drugs to take home with you (usually just a couple of weeks) and then you will have to see your own doctor for repeat prescriptions. You will be seen again in the hospital and they will ask you to exercise on a treadmill, while monitoring your heart, to see what effect any damage may have had on your exercise tolerance. You will probably be offered a cardiac rehabilitation programme where you will be able to ask questions about your individual recovery and will be told what to expect.

What are the complications of a heart attack?

The larger the heart attack and the longer before medical help was given, the greater the risk of complications, so if you had a small heart attack which was recognized quickly and treatment given, the chances are you will make a full recovery. Larger heart attacks are more likely to develop complications, especially if treatment was delayed for any reason. Complications include:

- heart failure, where the muscle is so damaged that the heart is no longer able to pump blood as effectively, leading to shortness of breath, sometimes on minimal exertion, and swollen ankles (see Chapter 7);
- rhythm problems, which are most likely to occur in the first few hours or days after a heart attack and are why your team will keep you in hospital under surveillance (see Chapter 8).

Once you have had one heart attack you are at increased risk of another at some point in the future, so it is vital that you address any lifestyle issues that put you at risk.

What is acute coronary syndrome?

You may hear this term during your stay in hospital and it is the term used to describe a range of conditions including heart attacks and **unstable angina**.

What is angina?

Angina usually occurs when the coronary arteries are narrowed by plaques. There is no total blockage but, because the arteries are narrower, the heart muscle can't get as much blood so when you are exercising, or even after eating a meal, your heart would normally pump more strongly to divert blood to the large muscles needed for exercise, or to the gut to aid digestion. If the blood supply is compromised then the heart muscle struggles and this presents as a pain across the chest, like that of a heart attack, but this pain should wear off if you rest. If you are diagnosed with angina, your doctor will discuss all the risk factors with you – these are the same as the ones for coronary heart disease – and you will be encouraged to address them. Your doctor will start you on medication to reduce your risk of heart attack and will give you a nitrate spray which you can spray under your tongue at the onset of an attack of angina. This is rapidly absorbed into the blood stream and will dilate the blood vessels. If angina lasts for more than 10 minutes, you should call an ambulance in case it is a heart attack. Angina can also less commonly be caused by spasm in the coronary artery walls. When it is predictable, angina can be described as stable. If you know that you are OK to walk around a supermarket, but would develop pain if you were to run for a bus, this is stable angina. If, however, the pain is triggered by less and less exertion, or even occurs while at rest, this is called unstable angina and should be considered a medical emergency as it could herald a heart attack.

Can I drive after a heart attack?

You should not drive for at least four weeks after a heart attack. If your recovery is going well, you should be fine to drive again at this stage but if you have had complications your doctors will advise you when driving becomes possible. If you have stable angina, you are safe to drive, but if you develop pains while driving you should stop immediately and, if your angina becomes unstable, you must stop driving until your symptoms are back under control.

How old is my heart?

Depending on your risk factors, your heart may actually be ageing faster than you. To find out your heart age, visit <www.nhs.uk/conditions/nhs-health-check/pages/check-your-heart-age-tool.aspx>

7

Heart failure

The heart is a muscular pump that pumps blood out from the ventricles to every part of the body. When the heart is healthy, a known volume of blood is ejected with each heartbeat. Heart failure is the term used to describe the situation when the heart is unable to pump so strongly. It may affect only the right ventricle, in which case it is called **right-sided heart failure**, or only the left, **left-sided heart failure**, or it can affect both ventricles. Heart failure may be due to an inability of the ventricular wall to stretch and allow enough blood to fill the ventricle during the resting phase, or diastole. This is called **diastolic heart failure**. Or it may be due to an inability of the ventricular wall to contract strongly during the pumping phase, systole, in which case it is called **systolic heart failure** – or it may be a combination of the two.

The most common cause of heart failure is coronary artery disease (or ischaemic heart disease) and this accounts for around 35–40 per cent of cases. High blood pressure is the cause of 15–20 per cent of cases and the remaining heart failure cases are due to problems with the heart muscle itself. These problems may occur out of the blue, or be due to alcohol, or some medication such as chemotherapy drugs. There may also be problems with the heart valves.

What are the symptoms of heart failure?

Heart failure makes you feel fatigued and tired. You may also feel nauseous and dizzy. Left-sided heart failure will make you feel short of breath on minimal exertion, such as walking up slopes. You may also feel short of breath when you lie down, and may wake in the night feeling very short of breath. Right-sided heart failure cause fluid retention, which means you are likely to have swollen ankles and legs and your liver may become enlarged. The severity of the symptoms depends on the degree of failure. So in mild heart failure, you may feel short of breath on walking. Severe heart failure will make you short of breath even at rest.

How is heart failure diagnosed?

If your doctor suspects heart failure from your description of your symptoms, he or she will feel your heart to see if it is enlarged and listen to the base of your lungs. If there is fluid on the lungs, he or she will hear crackles. Your doctor will also press a thumb into the skin of your ankle or lower leg. If this leaves a depression, that suggests fluid retention. And he or she will look at the blood vessels in your neck to see if there is an abnormal pulsation. If your doctor makes a diagnosis of heart failure, he or she will probably refer you to a specialist hospital heart failure service, as we know the outlook is better if you are looked after in this environment. They may arrange some of the tests below.

- *Blood tests* In particular they will check that you are not anaemic, and test your liver and kidney functions. They may test for cardiac enzymes, if they suspect a heart attack, and for a special protein that is released from the muscle wall of the atria when they are stretched; in heart failure the blood level of this protein is raised.
- *Chest X-ray* This will tell whether the heart is enlarged, and may also show if there is fluid on the lungs.
- *ECG* This is to check whether there is an abnormal rhythm that may have caused the heart failure, and will also show if the heart is strained.
- *Echocardiogram* This ultrasound test of the heart gives a

picture of the size of the heart, the size of each of the chambers and how they are functioning.

- *MRI* An MRI scan may be used to give a clearer picture of how your heart is working.
- *Cardiac biopsy* This may be done if the doctors suspect the failure is due to a problem with the heart muscle itself.

Is there anything I can do for myself?

It is important that you maintain a healthy weight, as it stands to reason that the heavier you are the more work your heart has to do just getting you around. If you smoke, you should stop straight away and your doctor will advise on local smoking cessation services to help you to quit. Unless your doctor advises against it, you should try to take regular exercise and stay as fit as you can. That may simply mean a daily walk around the block, but anything you can do to maintain your fitness will help your heart. Be careful about alcohol – drinking excessively can damage the heart muscle, and you don't want to do anything to cause any more damage, so women should stick to 14 units of alcohol a week and men should stick to 21 units, with at least two dry days each week.

I'm not usually a fan of weighing yourself too regularly but, if you have heart failure, it is good to get into the habit of weighing yourself each day. If you notice a sudden increase of several pounds, that is likely to be fluid not fat and you should see your doctor.

Your doctor will offer you the pneumococcal vaccination and a vaccination against influenza – make sure you accept these offers as you will be more prone to infection. You could also consider taking an omega-3 supplement as these have been shown to protect against symptoms worsening.

Will I need to take medication?

If you have symptoms you will need to take medication which may be a combination of the drugs listed below.

- *ACE inhibitors* These help regulate fluid in the body, and are thought to protect the heart, so slowing down the progression of the condition. They tend to drop blood pressure dramatically when they are first started, so your doctor may increase the dose gradually over a few weeks.
- *Diuretics* These work on the kidneys to help you pass more urine and remove the excess fluid that may have accumulated on your lungs or in your legs or liver. It is generally a good idea to take them in the morning, as if you take them later in the day you could find yourself up and down to the toilet at night.
- *Beta blockers* These slow down the heart rate and are thought to protect the heart from further deterioration.
- *Aldosterone receptor agonists* As with the ACE inhibitors, these work on an enzyme system in the kidney to help you remove excess fluid from your body.

You may also be on other medicines, such as aspirin, statins, and blood pressure pills or nitrates to treat coronary heart disease. It is important that you don't take Viagra or any similar drugs, as it can cause a dramatic drop in blood pressure if you have heart failure.

Will I need surgery?

Not all heart failure patients will need surgery, but if your doctor knows that you have coronary artery disease, you may need angioplasty to dilate the coronary arteries or even heart bypass surgery. If the heart failure is caused by valvular disease, you may need surgery to replace the damaged valve. If you have an underlying problem with heart rhythm, then you might be offered a pacemaker or a device that works as an automatic defibrillator and automatically gives your heart a shock if your rhythm goes too fast. In extreme cases, a heart transplant could be offered.

8

Heart rhythm problems

The heart is a muscular pump with an intricate wiring system that allows it to contract over 100,000 times a day without any conscious thought on our part. When the heart is healthy, those contractions are regular and strong and increase in rate when we are exercising, stressed or in pain.

The initial electrical impulse to signal a contraction starts in the right atrium, in an area referred to as the **sinoatrial** (or SA) node. This is like the heart's own natural pacemaker and it will fire off 60–80 times a minute in a healthy resting heart. The harder you exercise, the faster it produces these impulses. At its fastest, it will produce your maximum heart rate (MHR) – which is roughly 220 minus your age for men, and 210 minus your age for women. So if you are 40 and you are exercising as hard as you can the SA node will fire off 180 (220 – 40) times a minute.

Once triggered, the electrical impulse spreads across the atria causing the cardiac muscle in the atrial walls to contract, and this forces blood through one-way valves into the ventricles. Blood from the left atrium passes through the mitral valve into the left ventricle and blood from the right atria passes through the tricuspid valve into the right ventricle. The electrical impulse passes to the **atrioventricular** (AV) node between the atria and ventricles. From here there is a narrow pathway of electrical fibres called the **atrioventricular bundle**, which allows electrical activity to pass from the atria to the ventricles. The AV bundle splits into two branches known as the **Purkinje system** and, from here, the impulse spreads out across the ventricles causing them to contract and forcing blood out of two more one-way valves.

From the left ventricle, the blood passes through the aortic valve into the aorta and from the right ventricle, through the pulmonary valve into the pulmonary artery. When this process is working as it should the heart beats regularly at about 60–80 beats per minute at rest; this is called **sinus rhythm**. **Sinus bradycardia** refers to a situation where the heart beats more slowly, but still regularly, and this occurs in fit athletes, in some people while asleep and when the thyroid is underactive. **Sinus tachycardia** refers to the situation where the heart beats more frequently, say 100 beats per minute. Most commonly this might occur when you are exercising, are anxious or in pain. It can also occur when you have a fever, are anaemic or if your thyroid is overactive. It is normal to feel the occasional extra beat, particularly if you have been drinking a lot of caffeine or alcohol, and it doesn't necessarily mean there is a problem. These beats are referred to as **ectopic beats** and are rarely a sign of anything serious, but heart rates of less than 40 beats per minute, or more than 120 beats per minute, need investigating as does anyone with an irregular pulse. If an individual has an abnormal rate or rhythm to their heart this is called an **arrhythmia** and I will describe some types of arrhythmias below.

Supraventricular tachycardia

Supraventricular tachycardia (SVT) refers to a rapid heart rate (usually faster than 130 beats per minute and sometimes as fast as 250 beats per minute) that doesn't originate in the SA node. It starts in an area just above the ventricles (giving the term 'supra-ventricular') and passes straight to the ventricles, causing a rapid but regular heart beat. Sometimes these episodes are sporadic and short lived, and sometimes they can last for several hours and occur frequently. They can occur in healthy, young people. They may be triggered by caffeine or alcohol, so it is a good idea to cut back on these if this happens to you. Your doctor will want to confirm an SVT with an ECG tracing and, as your symptoms are likely to be intermittent, he or she may well need to do a 24-hour ECG to catch the rhythm. You might be able to correct an SVT by immersing your face in cold water, or by breathing in and then straining to breathe out but keeping your mouth closed and pinching your nose, as you would to pop your ears. If an SVT is prolonged and making you feel unwell with shortness of breath and dizziness, your doctor may suggest an electrical shock to the heart to revert the rhythm to sinus rhythm or a medicine into a vein. If you get frequent attacks, your doctor may prescribe medication to prevent them and in some cases an operation can be done, via a catheter inserted into the main vein in your groin, to remove the area where the abnormal electrical impulses arise.

Atrial fibrillation

In atrial fibrillation (AF) the atria don't contract regularly under the influence of the SA node. They fibrillate, causing an irregular pulse, which is often very fast. It occurs when the SA node is overridden by random electrical impulses from elsewhere in the atria. Some of these impulses pass through to the ventricles causing contraction of the ventricles in an irregular way. AF is very common – about 1 in 200 people over 40, and 1 in 10 over 80, have the condition. AF may occur in bouts, which resolve spontaneously without the need for treatment, but often recur. If an episode of AF resolves within a week it is referred to as **paroxysmal AF**. If it persists beyond seven days, then it is referred to as **persistent AF**.

What causes AF?

AF can be due a number of different conditions, some linked directly to the heart and some not. Cardiac related causes of AF include:

- hypertension (this is the most common cause of AF)
- coronary artery disease
- heart valve disease
- cardiomyopathies (diseases of the heart muscle)
- pericardial disease (disease of the tough outer layer protecting the heart).

In fact, any condition that puts a strain on the atria, or causes them to become enlarged, can cause AF. Non-cardiac causes of AF include:

- hyperthyroidism (overactive thyroid)
- excess alcohol
- excess caffeine
- obesity
- lung problems, including a blood clot on the lung, pneumonia or lung cancer.

How do I know if I have AF?

If you have slow AF, you may not be aware of a problem unless you physically take your pulse and notice that it is irregular. The more rapid the rate, the more likely you are to develop symptoms such as palpitations, shortness of breath, dizziness or chest pain. If you develop these symptoms, it is important that you get yourself checked out by your doctor.

What will my doctor do?

Your doctor will want to examine you, taking care to note the rate and rhythm of your pulse. If AF is suspected, he or she will arrange an ECG, which shows characteristic changes. Your doctor may also want to do blood tests to check you out for thyroid disease, and an echocardiogram, looking for the size and function of the heart chambers and for any problems with the valves.

Why does AF matter?

AF means that the heart doesn't pump efficiently and this can mean that blood flow becomes turbulent and clots can form. If these pass out of the heart into the brain they can block an artery and cause a stroke, which is why most people who have AF are offered medication to thin the blood and reduce the risk of stroke. Heart failure is also more common in AF, as the heart simply can't pump the blood as efficiently when the atria are fibrillating.

What other treatment will my doctor offer me?

If you are in fast AF, this makes your heart even less efficient and your doctor will want to control the rate with other medicines. The choice will depend on your individual circumstances and what other drugs you are on. Several different drugs can be used, including digoxin, beta blockers, and calcium channel blockers. If you are young (under 65), have only recently developed AF and have a structurally normal heart, your doctor may suggest referral for cardioversion with electric shock treatment. This is not very successful if you have enlarged heart chambers, damaged valves or have had AF for more than a year. If it is offered it has long-term success in about half of patients but about half will revert to AF. We can also use a medicine called **amiodarone** to revert the heart to a normal rhythm, but this has some long-term side effects such as fibrosis of the lungs, liver and thyroid problems. Occasionally it is possible to remove an area where the abnormal impulses are originating but this is not routine practice and is only available for very specific cases of AF.

Atrial flutter

Atrial flutter is similar to atrial fibrillation but less common and generally slower – typically someone in atrial flutter will have a heart rate of around 150 beats per minute. About a third of patients with flutter will also have AF and it is usually treated by removing an abnormal pathway rather than with medication.

Ventricular tachycardia

Ventricular tachycardia (VT) occurs when the electrical impulses in the ventricles become disrupted and override the normal rhythm. It often occurs after a heart attack and, if it lasts more than 30 seconds and is causing chest pain, shortness of breath or dizzy spells, it is a medical emergency which may need electrical shock treatment. There are also drugs, such as amiodarone, to treat VT. Some patients will need an implantable defibrillator, which is positioned under the skin near your collarbone, on your left-hand side. It monitors your heart rate, and if it detects VT, it will deliver an internal shock to revert the rhythm.

Ventricular fibrillation

Ventricular fibrillation is a medical emergency and usually occurs following a heart attack, but can occur in any situation where there is a lack of oxygen supply to the heart muscle. The patient is likely to collapse suddenly, and treatment is with electrical shock. Many public places now have defibrillators to deal with exactly this sort of emergency.

Heart block

All the rhythm disturbances I have discussed, up to this point, have meant a faster heart beat. In heart block, the heart is likely to beat more slowly. We talk about **first, second and third degree heart block**. First degree heart block occurs when there is a split second delay in the electrical impulses passing from the atria to the ventricles, and often has no symptoms but is picked up on a heart tracing. In second degree heart block there is increasing delay in the passage of impulses, which may result in symptoms such as light headedness or fainting. In third degree heart block, there is no passage of electrical impulse between the atria and the ventricles and the ventricles take over at a rate of about 40 beats per minute. This is likely to be associated with symptoms such as dizziness and fainting, and it also increases the risk of developing other rhythm problems. Mild degrees of heart block may require no treatment at all, but third degree heart block will usually require a pacemaker to be fitted to ensure your heart rate is fast enough.

9

Heart valve problems

There are four valves in the heart. On the left side, the mitral valve lies between the left atrium and left ventricle, and the aortic valve lies between the left ventricle and the aorta. On the right, the tricuspid valve lies between the right atrium and right ventricle, and the pulmonary valve lies between the right ventricle and the pulmonary artery. All the valves are designed to be one-way valves so when they are working well they prevent backflow of blood. I will describe each valve individually.

The mitral valve

The mitral valve lies between the left atrium and the left ventricle. It has two cusps and it is tethered by fibrous bands to the side of the ventricle that prevent it from turning inside out when the pressure in the ventricle rises, which occurs as the mitral valve contracts. Sometimes it can become leaky, which is called **mitral regurgitation**; sometimes it can becomes stiff and narrowed, which is called **mitral stenosis**.

Mitral regurgitation

Mitral regurgitation (MR) most commonly occurs as a process of ageing and the mitral valve stretching but it can also occur following a heart attack or as part of a disease of the heart muscle (see Chapter 10). In the past, it was much more common and was frequently due to an infection called **rheumatic fever**. Rheumatic fever is now rare in the developed world because of the availability of antibiotics. About 1 in 20 adults in the UK will have a floppy valve. It is particularly common in women and may cause no symptoms at all, only being picked up when a doctor listens to your heart. In fact that is exactly what happened to me – the first I knew that I had a floppy mitral valve was when my flatmate and I were practising for our final medical exams and she noticed I had a murmur!

How would I know if I have MR?

As I have said, if the regurgitation is mild you may have no idea you have the condition until a doctor examines your chest and notices a murmur. It is perfectly possible to go through life with MR and have no problems whatsoever. If the valve is very leaky though, it will allow significant amounts of blood back into the right atrium as the ventricle contracts, and this can ultimately cause the atrium to stretch and put a back pressure on to the vessels in the lungs. These changes may mean you experience palpitations, dizzy spells, shortness of breath, or even chest pain due to angina, as not enough blood is being pumped out of the aorta and into the coronary arteries. If the right atrium becomes stretched you are more prone to atrial fibrillation, which in turn increases your risk of a stroke. You could also develop heart failure. If the valve is damaged, it can be more prone to infection and you may need antibiotics to cover, for example, dental work to prevent bugs from your mouth entering the blood stream and colonizing on the damaged valve. This is generally only necessary if you have an infection at the time of the procedure.

What will my doctor do?

If your doctor notices a murmur during systole (the contraction of the ventricles) he or she will suggest that you have an echocardiogram, which will show if the valve is leaking. Depending on the severity of the leak, he or she will then advise on whether further action is needed. Most people won't require surgery to repair or replace the valve, but many will need medication to treat the complications such as heart failure or atrial fibrillation.

Mitral stenosis

Mitral stenosis (MS) is when the mitral valve becomes stiff or narrowed and doesn't open properly, meaning less blood can leave the atria during atrial contraction. This, in turn means less blood arrives in the ventricles. The atria have to work harder and harder to push blood through the narrowed valve, and this can lead to thickening of the muscle wall, which we call **hypertrophy**. Ultimately, it can also lead to back pressure in the veins in the lungs that drain into the right atrium.

How would I know if I have MS?

Just like MR, if the stenosis is mild you may have no symptoms at all, but as the narrowing worsens you may notice increasing shortness of breath on less and less exertion. You may develop angina, if insufficient blood is leaving the left ventricle in the aorta and supplying the coronary arteries. If your lungs become congested, you may cough up blood-stained sputum and you will be more prone to atrial fibrillation and heart failure as the right atrial chamber enlarges.

What will my doctor do?

There are certain signs that your doctor will look out for if he or she suspects MS. These include flushed cheeks and, in severe cases, a blue tinge to the lips. Your liver may be enlarged due to congestion, and the veins in your neck may appear engorged. Your doctor will confirm the diagnosis with an ultrasound test of your heart. If you are diagnosed with MS, your doctor will advise on what medications are needed, and these will depend on the severity of your symptoms and which complications you develop. There are a number of surgical options available to more severe cases and these include the following.

- *Mitral valve stretch* This is done using a balloon, which is inserted via a catheter into the large blood vessel in your groin using X-ray control. It is then guided into position in the valve, and the balloon is inflated to open the narrowed valve.
- *Mitral valve repair* This is a more major procedure and involves open heart surgery where the edges of the valves are trimmed back to open the valve.
- *Mitral valve replacement* This is another open heart surgery technique. A mechanical valve or an animal valve (usually from a pig) can be used to replace the damaged valve. If you have a mechanical valve, you may be aware of a funny clicking sound as it shuts with each heart beat.

Aortic valve

The aortic valve lies between the top of the left ventricle and the bottom of the aorta. It has three cusps. Just like the mitral valve it can become leaky (**aortic regurgitation**) or narrowed (**aortic stenosis**).

Aortic regurgitation

Aortic regurgitation (AR) occurs when the valve doesn't close properly after blood has been pumped out of the ventricle into the aorta, meaning that blood can flow back into the ventricle and doesn't get pumped around the body. It used to be much more common as it is also linked to rheumatic fever. Today it can sometimes be a problem that a child is born with, or it can be linked to a number of conditions which affect the tissue at the base of the aorta, allowing it to widen so that the cusps no longer meet tightly. These conditions include rheumatoid arthritis, Marfan's syndrome, Reiter's syndrome and syphilis.

How would I know if I have AR?

A small leak is likely to go unnoticed and the first you may know about it is if a doctor hears a heart murmur when he or she is examining your heart. If the regurgitation becomes more severe, you may become dizzy, or develop angina, as not enough blood is being pumped into the aorta. If things progress further, you may develop heart failure.

What will my doctor do?

If your doctor suspects AR, he or she will arrange an echocardiogram to assess how the valve and the heart are functioning. Your doctor will give you medication to treat any of the complications, such as angina or heart failure. You may be offered antibiotics to prevent bacteria infecting the damaged valve if you have, for example, a dental procedure. We used to do this routinely, but now we only generally give antibiotics if you have an infection at the time of the procedure. If you need surgery, your specialist will suggest that you have the valve replaced before there is too much damage to your heart.

Tricuspid valve

The tricuspid valve, as its name suggests, has three cusps and lies between the right atrium and the right ventricle. Disease of the tricuspid valve is much less common than diseases of the mitral or aortic valves.

Tricuspid regurgitation

Tricuspid regurgitation (TR) is rarely a problem that occurs on its own; it is usually associated with a back pressure from right-sided heart problems.

How would I know I have TR?

It is estimated that about 1 in 100 people have a minor degree of TR but with no symptoms and no consequences. Significant TR is often associated with other problems and may make you short of breath and fatigued. You notice discomfort in the upper right side of your abdomen, as your liver may be engorged, and you may notice a blue tinge to your lips.

What will my doctor do?

Your doctor will examine your heart, listening for a characteristic murmur. Your doctor will check the veins in your neck, as these may be engorged and showing abnormal pulsations, and he or she will check your abdomen for an enlarged liver. If TR is suspected he or she will arrange an echocardiogram. Your doctor will treat any complications such as heart failure appropriately and, as the condition progresses, he or she may refer you for valve replacement surgery.

Tricuspid stenosis

As with MS, tricuspid stenosis (TS) refers to narrowing of the tricuspid valve and, since this occurs almost exclusively due to complications of rheumatic fever, it is now very rare in the western world. It is also almost always associated with problems with other valves.

How would I know if I have TS?

TS may make you feel fatigued, short of breath and cold. You may also have a loss of appetite and discomfort in your abdomen and a blue tinge to your lips.

What will my doctor do?

Your doctor will examine you, as he or she would for the other valve problems, and arrange an echocardiogram. Your doctor will treat any other complications and if you do need surgery, it is likely, as other valves are usually involved, that you will need open heart surgery and your specialist will probably want to operate on all the damaged valves at the same time.

Pulmonary valve

The pulmonary valve lies between the right ventricle and the pulmonary artery. It has three cusps. Pulmonary valve disease is usually due to congenital heart disease, but it can be associated with infection or other conditions such as Marfan's syndrome, or carcinoid or pulmonary hypertension. Just like all the other valves, the pulmonary valve can be leaky or narrowed.

Pulmonary regurgitation

Pulmonary regurgitation is generally well-tolerated and tends not to have much in the way of symptoms, unless it is very severe. It may, over years, lead to dilation of the right ventricle and impaired function, which can cause shortness of breath on exertion. In severe cases patients can develop ventricular tachycardia, and pulmonary regurgitation can be the cause of sudden death.

Valve surgery is only undertaken if symptoms develop or there is known right ventricular dilation. In extreme cases, where severe right-sided heart failure develops, a heart–lung transplant may be the only option.

Pulmonary stenosis

Pulmonary stenosis tends to be a congenital problem and may even be diagnosed, antenatally, in the womb. The symptoms will depend very much on the severity of the narrowing, but include shortness of breath, dizzy spells and fainting. Once diagnosed, the specialists will decide on which surgical procedure to perform to prevent the development of right-sided heart failure in early life.

10

Heart muscle disorders

In this chapter, I will discuss the cardiomyopathies – *cardio* (heart)-*myo* (muscle)-*pathy* (abnormality). They can affect people of all ages and most are inherited but, although not curable, patients can expect to live a full and long life with the correct treatment. There are several different types.

Hypertrophic cardiomyopathy

Hypertrophic cardiomyopathy (HOCM) is an inherited condition where the muscle in the heart wall becomes thickened, which can be seen on an echocardiogram. It is caused by a change in one or more genes so, if you have HOCM, your children will have a 50 per cent chance of inheriting the condition. It is much more common than people realize, affecting 1 in 500 people in the UK. Some will have very little in the way of symptoms, but when the heart wall becomes thick it also becomes stiff and symptoms may develop as the heart becomes less efficient at pumping blood around the body. Symptoms may include any of the following – pain in the chest, shortness of breath, palpitations, dizziness or fainting. What symptoms you develop, and how severe they are, will depend on which part of the heart muscle is affected and how badly. People with HOCM may also develop heart rhythm problems. Very rarely, people with HOCM can develop a life-threatening rhythm problem and if your doctor thinks you are at increased risk, he or she may suggest you have an implantable defibrillator fitted. Many people with HOCM will need no treatment at all, but if you are prone to rhythm problems, your doctor may suggest medication or a pacemaker if your rhythm tends to be slow. You should be able to lead a normal life with HOCM, although you may be advised against physically demanding sports and careers. You can drive with HOCM but you would not be able to take your HGV licence or drive a commercial passenger vehicle.

Dilated cardiomyopathy

Dilated cardiomyopathy (DCM) patients have the opposite problem to HOCM patients as in DCM the heart muscle becomes dilated and thin, which can be seen clearly on an echocardiogram. It particularly affects the left ventricle. DCM can also be inherited and, again, if you have DCM, your children will have a 50 per cent chance of having the condition. It can also be caused by excess alcohol, viral infections, uncontrolled high blood pressure and heart valve problems. If it occurs as a result of these then it is unlikely that it will be passed on to any children.

Because the left ventricle is dilated in DCM, and the muscle wall thin, it means that the left ventricle is unable to pump blood around the body as efficiently and people with DCM are prone to heart failure, meaning they feel fatigued, short of breath on minimal exertion and have palpitations or swollen ankles from fluid retention. Just like HOCM, the treatment will depend on the severity of the symptoms and any complications that develop so it could include medication, an implantable defibrillator or a pacemaker. And, similarly, you may be advised to avoid high impact sports and will not be allowed to take your HGV driving test or drive a commercial passenger vehicle.

Arrhythmogenic right ventricular cardiomyopathy

Arrythmogenic right ventricular cardiomyopathy (ARVC) is also an inherited condition, although it is not inherited in the same way as HOCM and DCM. In fact, it is possible to inherit the mutated gene but not develop the condition. In ARVC the heart muscle fibres are not held together properly. Normally heart muscle cells are bound together by proteins, but in ARVC these proteins are not fully developed, which means the muscle fibres are not bound together so well and fatty deposits can accumulate between the muscle fibres. This can occur anywhere in the heart but most commonly it affects the right ventricle, which becomes stretched and less efficient. It can also spread to affect the left ventricle. In the early stages there may be no symptoms at all. If it progresses (and it doesn't always) people can be prone to problems with rhythm disturbances. In some instances, patients go on to develop right-sided heart failure and, ultimately, left-sided heart failure.

Takotsubo cardiomyopathy

Unlike the cardiomyopathies discussed above, takotsubo cardiomyopathy (also called **stress cardiomyopathy**) is a temporary condition. The word *takotsubo* is Japanese for 'octopus pot', and the condition got its name because the heart becomes a similar shape with a narrow neck and a round bottom. We don't really know why it happens, but it does seem to be linked to extreme emotional distress. It has in the past even been referred to as 'broken heart syndrome'. The good news is that it is completely reversible, usually over a period of days or weeks, and doesn't tend to recur.

Primary restrictive non-hypertrophic cardiomyopathy

Primary restrictive non-hypertrophic cardiomyopathy is a rare condition where the atria are enlarged and the ventricles may be small. It is associated with other conditions such as:

- *amyloidosis*, a condition where abnormal deposits of a protein called amyloid are deposited in the organs of the body;
- *sarcoidosis*, a condition where red, swollen pieces of tissue, called **granulomas**, are deposited in the organs of the body;
- *endocarditis*, a rare infection of the heart.

It can cause right-sided heart failure, and treatment is of the symptoms. In extreme cases, heart transplant is the only option.

Peripartum cardiomyopathy

Peripartum cardiomyopathy is rare and affects women in the last trimester of pregnancy, or within five months of delivery. It is more common in obese women who have had several pregnancies and are over 30 years old. Nearly half of all patients make a full recovery within six months.

Tachycardia cardiomyopathy

Prolonged periods of tachycardia can lead to dilation of the heart chambers resulting in tachycardia cardiomyopathy, a clinical condition similar to dilated cardiomyopathy.

11

Arterial problems

Abdominal aortic aneurysm

The aorta is the main artery leaving the left ventricle. It arches up into the chest and then down through the diaphragm into the abdomen, where it divides into the iliac arteries in the pelvis. It is the largest artery in the body and, in slim people, it can be felt pulsating in the abdomen. Sometimes it becomes dilated and is at risk of rupture. I remember, as a junior doctor, rushing to theatre on many an occasion with a patient with a ruptured abdominal aortic aneurysm. Sadly, many of those patients didn't survive, which is why we now have a screening programme in the UK for all men over the age of 65. We only screen men because aortic aneurysms are much more common in men. The test involves an ultrasound to measure the diameter of the aorta. A healthy aorta should be about 2 cm in diameter. If it is more than 3 cm, this is defined as an aneurysm and once formed it is only likely to get bigger. The more dilated the aorta is, the greater the chance of spontaneous rupture. As a rough guide, an aortic aneurysm of 5 cm has a 1 per cent chance of rupturing per year, while an aneur--ysm of 8 cm has a 50 per cent chance of rupture per year.

How would I know if I have an abdominal aortic aneurysm?

More often than not, unless you have been screened, you probably wouldn't have a clue because the dilation itself doesn't cause any symptoms until it is large enough to cause a pressure effect, when it may cause you some back pain. If the aneurysm ruptures, you will experience severe abdominal and/or back pain and will collapse and lose consciousness very quickly due to huge blood loss.

Why do aneurysms form?

There is no one cause for an aneurysm forming. They are four times as common in men as they are in women and are extremely rare under the age of 60. Other risk factors include a family history, so if your mother or father had an aneurysm, you are at higher risk. They are also more common in smokers and in anyone who has an increased risk of vascular disease in general, which means diabetics, people with high blood pressure or high cholesterol, the very overweight and those who do very little exercise. Very rarely an aneurysm forms in younger people without these risk factors, and that is thought to be due to an inherited condition where the elasticity of the aortic wall is impaired.

What tests will my doctor do?

If you are male, over 65 and registered with an NHS GP, you will automatically be called for a screening ultrasound. This is totally painless. The radiographer will simply put some jelly on your abdomen and, using an ultrasound probe, will be able to measure the diameter of your aorta. The walls of the aorta will show up as white lines and the blood will look black. The whole test takes about 10 minutes and you will be given the results straight away. Like all screening tests available on the NHS, I would encourage you to attend. The NHS is not awash with cash and if it is offering you a test, it must think it is worth it! It is hoped that screening for abdominal aortic aneurysms could reduce death from rupture by as much as 50 per cent. That seems a no-brainer to me, so when you get your call, make sure you go!

If you have an aneurysm you will probably be called back for regular ultrasound tests. If it is larger than 5.5 cm, your doctor will refer you to a vascular surgeon to discuss surgery.

You may also be asked to go for a CT scan to check whether the aneurysm involves any of the arteries that branch off of the aorta, as this has implications for surgery.

Will I definitely need surgery?

No. Smaller aneurysms aren't usually operated on because this is major surgery with its own risks. If your aneurysm is less than 5.5 cm in diameter, there is a 1 per cent risk of rupture but the surgery to repair it has a greater risk of death, so your doctor will monitor you with regular ultrasounds. The decision on whether to operate will depend on the size of your aneurysm, your state of health and your wishes. So this is definitely not a 'one size fits all' kind of decision.

What does the surgery involve?

The traditional operation involves an incision down the midline of your tummy. The diseased part of the aorta is removed and replaced with a graft, which is stitched in place. There is also a newer technique which involves inserting a tube into the major artery in the groin and passing it up through the diseased part of the aorta. It is then clipped into place and forms a new aortic passage. This is called an **endovascular repair** and is a more minor procedure, but has the disadvantage of possibly needing to be repeated in the future, while a graft usually lasts for life.

What can I do to reduce my risk of developing an aortic aneurysm?

Anything you can do to reduce your cardiovascular risk will improve your outlook. So if you smoke, stop now! Your doctor will be able to help you with information about local smoking cessation services. Try to maintain a healthy weight (BMI between 18.5 and 25) and take regular exercise – at least 30 minutes five times a week. Eat a healthy, well-balanced diet and make sure you know your blood pressure and cholesterol level. You really don't know what these are unless you have them measured and you could be sitting on a time bomb if you don't get them checked. If your doctor finds that either of these are raised, he or she will advise on treatment.

Berry aneurysms

These are found in the arteries supplying the brain. They look like a ballooning of the blood vessel on one side. The ballooned area is weaker and prone to spontaneous rupture.

How would I know if I have a berry aneurysm?

You probably wouldn't. They don't cause any symptoms until they rupture. When they start to leak, they classically cause a severe headache. People say it is like being kicked in the head. If you experience a headache like this it is important that you seek urgent medical help. If the doctor suspects an aneurysm, he or she will arrange an urgent CT or MRI of your head. If you have a close relative who has had a berry aneurysm, you may be at increased risk and should discuss with your doctor as to whether you need a scan. People with polycystic kidneys, coarctation of the aorta (a birth defect where the first part of the aorta is narrowed) or endocarditis, an infection of the heart, are also at increased risk.

What will happen if the aneurysm bursts?

Sadly, if the aneurysm bursts there is a risk you won't survive. At medical school we were always taught the rule of thirds. If a berry aneurysm bursts, a third of people make a full recovery, a third survive with some disability, and a third don't make it.

Can an aneurysm be repaired?

Yes. There are two main techniques. Either the aneurysm can be clipped via a hole in the skull called a **craniotomy** or an endovascular technique can be used to seal off the aneurysm. The decision on whether to have surgery, will depend on the size of your aneurysm (the larger the aneurysm, the greater the risk of rupture), your general health and your wishes. It is vital that you are aware of the risks and possible complications before making your decision.

Peripheral vascular disease

If the peripheral arteries, most commonly those supplying the legs, become narrowed they can cause claudication and even gangrene.

What is claudication?

Claudication is a severe pain, like cramp, that occurs in the lower leg when walking. It is caused by not enough blood being supplied to the muscles in the leg, which is usually due to narrowing of the blood vessels with atheroma. It can sometimes be caused by spasm in the blood vessels. The more narrow the arteries, the more compromised the blood flow and the less distance you will be able to walk before the symptoms begin. If you rest, the pain resolves but recurs again when you start to exercise. If nothing is done about it, and the narrowing in the blood vessels is allowed to progress, then eventually the pain becomes constant even at rest and, ultimately, if the blood flow is severely compromised, gangrene develops.

Who gets claudication?

Claudication is more common in men than women and is rare under the age of 60. It is much more common in smokers, in anyone who has established coronary artery disease and those with other cardiac risk factors, such as high blood pressure, high cholesterol, diabetes and obesity.

What will my doctor do?

If your doctor suspects claudication he or she will first want to take your blood pressure and feel the pulses in your legs. Your doctor may check the blood pressure in your arm as normal, and then also in your lower leg. Your doctor is looking for a difference in the two pressures, suggesting a problem with blood flow. Your doctor may press your big toe, which should blanch under pressure. In healthy individuals, the colour should return quickly, but in those with poor blood supply it can take some time before the skin returns to its normal colour. Your doctor will then want to do some tests, starting with blood tests to check you for diabetes and high cholesterol, and will arrange an ultrasound to look at the blood flow in your legs. Your doctor may also arrange a CT scan, or a magnetic resonance angiography, to have a more detailed look at the blood flow in your legs.

What can I do to help myself?

Preventing claudication from progressing is all about managing cardiovascular risk factors. So if you smoke, you should try to stop straight away. Maintain a healthy weight and try to get what exercise you can. Eat a healthy, well-balanced diet. It is important that you manage high blood pressure and diabetes too, and your doctor may advise you to take blood thinning drugs, such as aspirin, to improve flow.

Is there anything else that can be done?

As well as managing any underlying risk factors, your doctor may prescribe drugs to help dilate the arteries or reduce the stickiness of blood. If these aren't enough to relieve symptoms, you may be referred for a surgical procedure. There are several options including:

- *angioplasty*, where a balloon is inserted into the narrowed area and blown up to help dilate the artery;
- *stenting*, where a mesh is placed inside the artery to help keep it open;
- *grafting*, where a piece of your own vein, or synthetic graft, is used to replace the narrowed vessel.

12

Venous problems

As I mentioned in the first chapter, veins have thinner walls than arteries, as the blood is under much lower pressure after having passed through the capillary bed. The larger veins have one-way valves in them to prevent blood from sinking back with gravity and pooling in the lower leg. There are superficial veins that lie just below the skin, and deep leg veins that pass through the muscles, and they are connected to each other by small veins called perforators.

Varicose veins

Varicose veins are the bumpy veins that look prominent in the legs and are caused by back pressure. If this pressure causes the valves to fail then more pressure is placed on the valves below, and it is easy to see how the problem gets worse and worse.

Who gets varicose veins?

Varicose veins are more common in women than men, and they are more common the older we get. They are also more common in people who are overweight, pregnant women and in people who stand still for long periods of time.

What can I do to help varicose veins?

Once varicose veins have formed they won't go away without treatment but you can prevent them getting worse by maintaining a healthy weight and being as active as possible. If your job involves lots of standing, try to move on the spot as much as you can even if it is just rocking back-wards and forwards on your heels. This movement squeezes the muscles in your calves, which encourages blood flow back towards the heart. Wear compression stockings when-ever you can, and when you get home try to put your feet up as much as you can. Ideally, your feet should be higher than your heart so invest in a footstool to use when you are watching television, and rest your feet on that, preferably with some cushions underneath. At night, rest your feet on a pillow in bed.

Do I need any other treatment?

If it is just the appearance of your veins that you don't like, I'm afraid you are unlikely to get any specific treat-ment for them on the NHS, as this is deemed a purely cosmetic problem. If, however, they cause you pain or you are developing varicose eczema, your doctor can refer you for assessment. Varicose eczema is dry, itchy skin usually around the ankle, which sometimes also looks discoloured. This can lead to ulceration if left untreated. It is important that you use plenty of moisturizer to keep the skin well hydrated. Your doctor will arrange a special ultrasound test to look at the flow and decide what treatment you should have.

What operations can be done?

In the past, we used to tie off the perforator veins and then pull the diseased vein out through an incision in the groin. The legs were then firmly bandaged and patients were asked to do lots of walking during the recovery period. This pro-cedure is still done today but only when newer techniques have been tried first. These techniques include:

- *laser treatment*, to heat up the vein and seal it;
- *radiofrequency ablation*, which uses heat to shrivel the vein;

- *sclerotherapy*, where a special foam is injected into the veins to cause them to shrink.

Deep vein thrombosis

Deep vein thromboses are blood clots that form in the deep veins of the legs. In the UK, 1 in 1000 people develop a deep vein thrombosis (DVT) each year.

Who gets DVTs?

Anyone can get a DVT, but there are a number of risk factors which would make a DVT more likely. These include:

- a previous DVT
- obesity
- inactivity
- a family history of blood clots
- smoking
- dehydration
- long-haul flights
- long hospital stays
- pregnancy
- some medicines, including the combined contraceptive pill
- cancer
- heart and lung disease
- Hughes syndrome, a condition associated with sticky blood and recurrent miscarriage
- thrombophilia, a genetic condition associated with a predisposition to clotting.

How would I know if I have a DVT?

A DVT will cause your leg to become swollen and painful. It will be tender to the touch, and may feel warm and look red. The pain may be worse if you flex your foot up towards your shin. If you have any doubt, it is important that you get it checked out, as if left untreated a piece of the clot could break away and become lodged in the vessels supplying the lungs. This is called a **pulmonary embolus** (or PE) and is potentially fatal.

What will my doctor do?

Your doctor will examine your leg and, if he or she suspects a DVT, may take a blood test looking for something called **D-dimers**. These are breakdown products of a blood clot and are often raised in the presence of a DVT. Your doctor may also refer you for a special form of ultrasound, called a Doppler, which looks at blood flow in the veins.

What treatment will I need?

You will be prescribed medication to thin the blood and prevent the clot from enlarging. The most common treatment is a drug called **warfarin**, but it can take a few days to work so you will be taught how to inject yourself with another medication while you are waiting for it to work. People react very differently to warfarin so you will need regular blood tests to check how you are responding and to fine tune your dose. You will usually have to take warfarin for between three and six months but your doctor will advise on your individual case. You will probably be asked to wear compression stockings, as these reduce the risk of recurrence and of developing what is called **post-thrombotic syndrome**. This is where there is ongoing pain and swelling at the site, often with discolouration of the skin and sometimes with associated ulceration.

How can I reduce my risk of DVT?

You can reduce your risk of DVT by stopping smoking, maintaining a healthy weight and being as mobile as possible. Avoid sitting still for long periods and try not to sit with your legs crossed. If your job involves you being sedentary, try to rock your feet back and forth, or draw circles in the air with your feet, to keep the blood pumping around. If you are travelling long distances, try to walk up and down the plane every hour. Drink plenty of water, but not alcohol as this can predispose to dehydration.

Index